HOME REMEDIES FOR EAR, NOSE AND THROAT DISORDERS, AN EASY GUIDE

BY YUORZEGH EZEKIEL (ENT NURSE PRACTIONER)

INTRODUCTION

Ear, nose and throat conditions are part of the nagging health problems globally. According to the World Health Organization (WHO), 2.5 billion people are projected to have some degree of hearing loss by 2050 and at least 700 will require hearing rehabilitation. Over 1 billion young adults are at risk of permanent, avoidable hearing loss due to unsafe listening practices.

This book serves as an easy guide for managing some ear, nose and throat conditions outside the health facility setting. It also highlight some effective ways to prevent ear, nose and throat diseases.

CHAPTERS

FIRST AID MANAGEMENT OF NASAL BLEEDING

1. Sit up and lean slightly forward. By remaining upright you reduce blood pressure in the veins of your nose. This discourages further bleeding and also help you avoid swallowing of blood.

2. Gently your blow nose to remove blood clot.

3. Use your thumb and index finger to pinch the anterior (soft) part of your nostrils shut and breathe through your mouth.

4. Continue to pinch for 10 to 15 minutes. Pinching sends pressure to the bleeding point on the nasal septum and often stops the flow of blood.

5. To avoid re-bleeding, don't pick or blow your nose and don't bend down for several hours.

6. Keep lead higher than the level of your heart. You can also gently apply petroleum jelly to the inside of your nose using cotton swab.

7. Apply ice pack to the bridge of your nose if bleeding continues or apply adrenaline to a piece of gauze and pack the bleeding nose.

8. If re-bleeding occurs, consult your doctor.

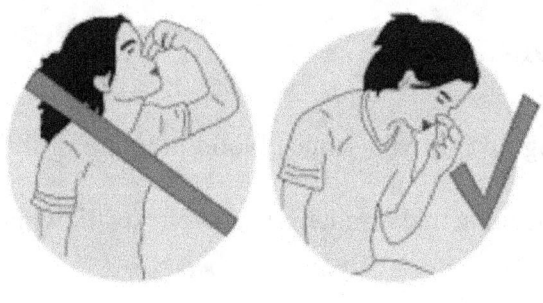
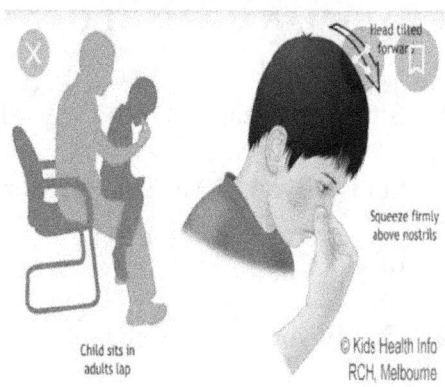

When to seek emergency care

➤ The bleeding last for more than 30 minutes.

➤ You feel faint or lightheaded.

➤ The bleed follows an accident, a fall or an injury to your head, including a punch in the face that may have broken your nose.

NOTE: consult your doctor if you experience frequent nose bleeds or have nasal bleeding after taking blood thinners such aspirin or warfarin.

TEN SIMPLE WAYS TO PRETECT YOUR EARS

I. Avoid using cotton swabs to clean your ears. Your ears usually do a good job cleaning themselves and don't need extra care.

II. Avoid using foreign objects such as matchsticks, keys, feathers etc into your ears. This may traumatize your ear canal/eardrum and cause ear pain.

III. Do not allow water to enter your ears. This will increase the PH of wax in your ears resulting in external ear infection.

IV.   Use ear plugs when you are around loud noises.

V.   Turn the volume down when listening to your radio, television set or using mobile phone.

VI.   If you are exposed to loud noises for prolong period of time, like at a concert, bar or stadium, your ears will need time to recover. You can sleep outside for 5 minutes every so often in order to let the ears rest.

VII.   Check your ears regularly.

VIII.   Manage stress.

IX.   Take medications only as directed by your doctor or ENT nurse practitioner.

X.   Consult your doctor or ENT nurse practitioner if you have ear pain, itching, fullness or ear discharge.

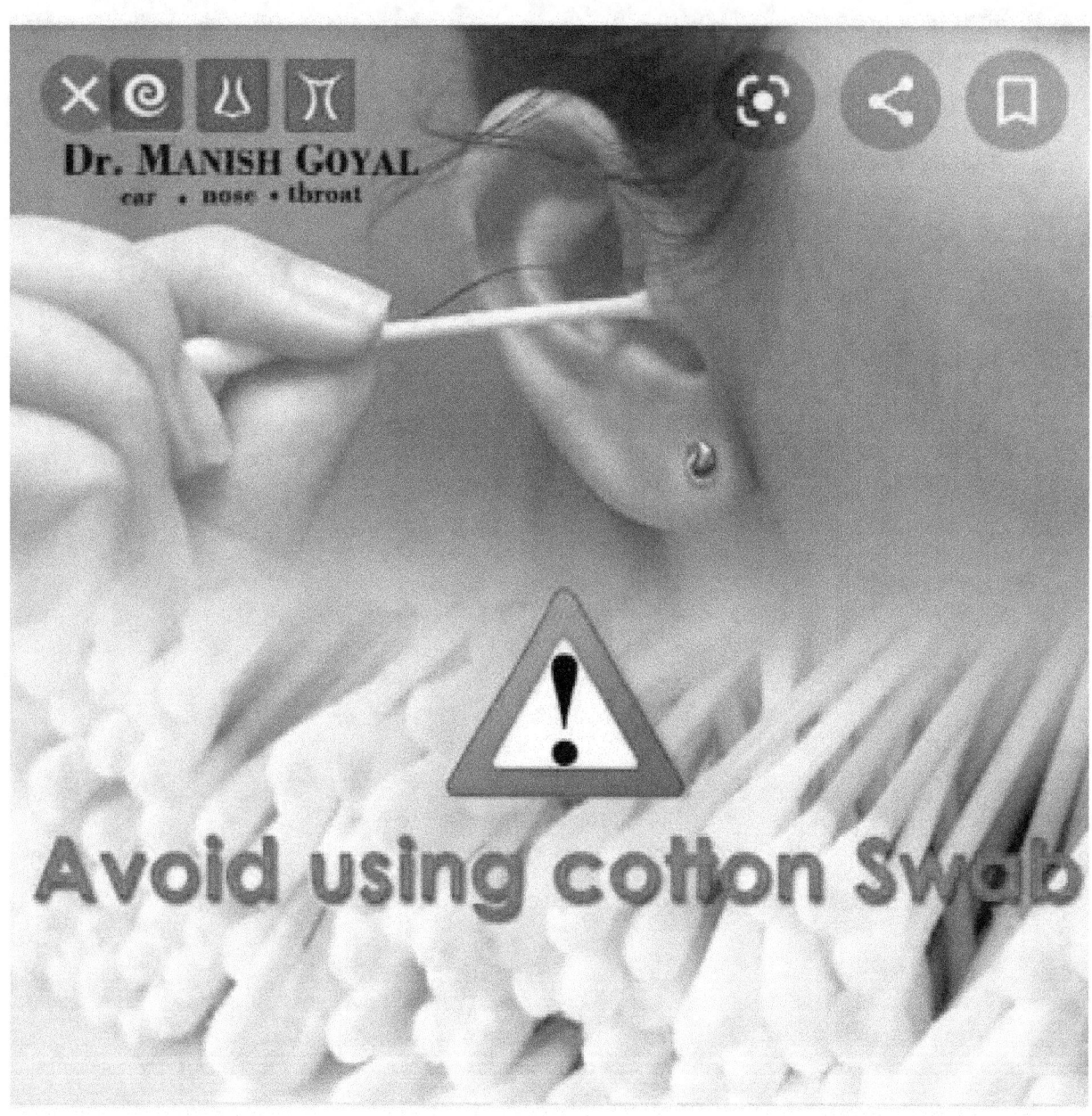

OTITIS MEDIA

Definition: Otitis media is the inflammation of the middle ear. It is caused by bacteria or viruses. This infection often result from another illness such as cold or allergy. This produces symptoms such as ear pain, fever, pulling of ears, crying and trouble sleeping.

HOW TO PREVENT OTITIS MEDIA IN CHILDREN

- ❖ Avoid giving your infant a pacifier.
- ❖ Breastfeed infants instead of bottle feeding if possible. Infants should be breastfed with head upright not in a lying down position.
- ❖ Get your child vaccinated against seasonal flu and pneumococcus.
- ❖ Consult your doctor if your child allergic to certain substances.
- ❖ Consult your doctor if your child suffers frequent upper respiratory tract infections, breaths through the mouth or snores when sleeping. That could be a sign of enlarged adenoids.

SIMPLE WAYS TO MAINTAIN VOCAL HYGIENE

- ✓ Stay hydrated.
- ✓ Compensate for dehydrating agents.
- ✓ Reduce high intensity voice use (voice abuse).
- ✓ Limit smoke inhalation.
- ✓ Control allergen exposure.
- ✓ Manage acid reflux.
- ✓ Consult your physician if you have voice problems.

VOCAL HYGIENE GUIDELINES

PRISMATIC
SPEECH SERVICES

1 Stay Hydrated!

If you're not sure how hydrated you are, check the color of your urine.

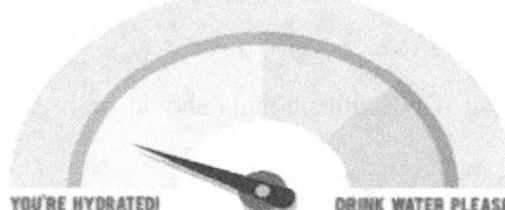

YOU'RE HYDRATED!   DRINK WATER PLEASE!

2 Compensate for Dehydrating Agents

All of these tend to make one lose water quicker than one drinks; however, how much water one loses is different from person to person. If one or more of these factors is present in your life, consider drinking more water to compensate.

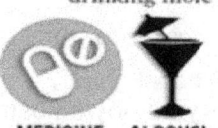
MEDICINE   ALCOHOL   ARID CLIMATE   EXERCISE

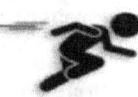

3 Reduce High Intensity Voice Use

Prolonged talking, screaming, yelling, chronic coughing or throat clearing all can cause nodules, polyps or cysts to form on the vocal folds.

4 Limit Smoke Inhalation

Both direct smoke inhalation and secondhand smoking cause dehydration and permanent damage to the larynx, lungs, and mouth.

5 Control Allergen Exposure

Both allergens and many allergy medications can affect one's ability to produce a clear, healthy sound. Research and discuss with your doctor to find the least dehydrating medication which works for you.

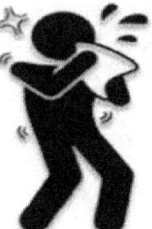

6 Manage Reflux

Reflux is when stomach acid leaks up the esophagus and on to the vocal folds. This exposure to caustic acid can cause or increase vocal fold damage. Discuss treatment with your speech-language pathologist or primary care physician.

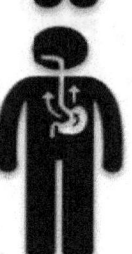

SIMPLE WAYS OF MAINTAINING NASAL AND SINUS HYGIENE

- Practice frequent hand washing and avoid inserting your fingers into your nose.

- Avoid people infected with common cold or influenza.

- Nasal irrigation with saline solution or steam inhalation can help decongest your nose and sinus and clear excess mucus in the nose and sinuses.

- Drink 8-10 glasses of water each day to stay hydrated and keep your nasal pathway moist.

- Avoid alcohol and caffeinated beverages (they can cause fluid loss and dehydration)

- If you are using humidifier or vaporizer, clean it regularly to prevent mould build-up.

- Exercise daily.

- Eat a balance diet with supplemental vitamins, especially vitamin c.

- Stop smoking and /or avoid tobacco.

- Sleep with your head elevated 30°C

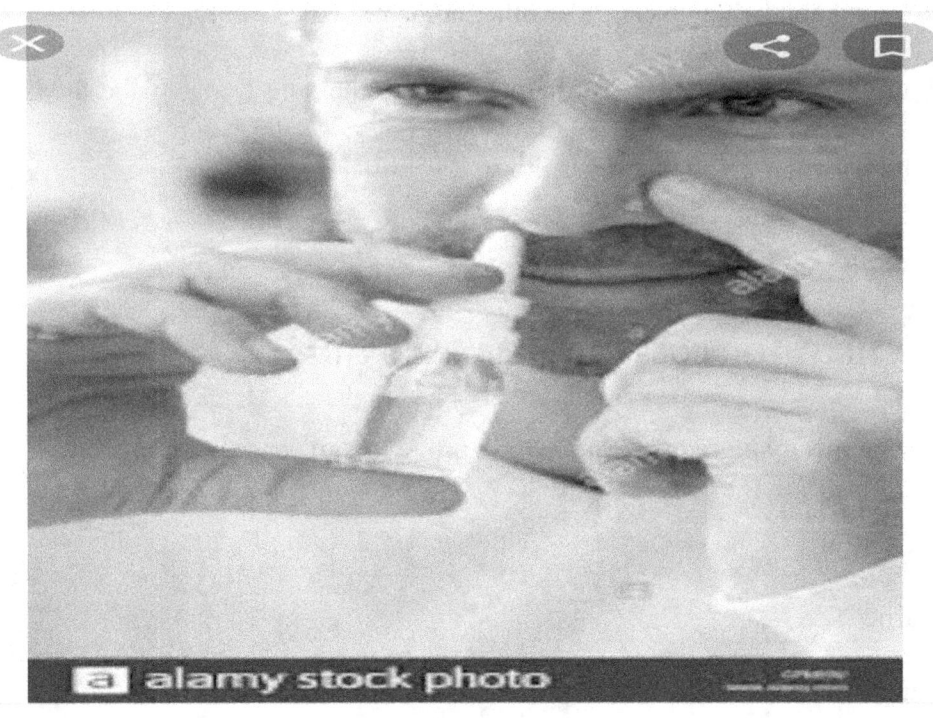

HOME REMEDIES FOR TONSILITIS

- Salt water gaggling; Gaggling and rinsing with salt water can help sooth a sore throat and pain caused by tonsillitis. It can also reduce inflammation and may even help to treat the infection. Stir half tea spoons of salt in 4 ounces of warm water, make sure the salt is completely dissolved then, gaggle swish through the mouth for several seconds spit it out.

- Licorice lozenges; Lozenges can help to soothe the throat. Lozenges containing licorice as an ingredient can have a strong anti-inflammatory benefits. Lozenges should not be given to young children due to choking risk. Throat sprays should be used instead.

- Warm tea with raw honey; Warm beverages like tea can help to reduce discomfort that can occur as a result of tonsillitis. Raw honey has strong antibacterial properties and help to treat the infection causing the tonsillitis.

- Popsicles and ice chips; Cold can be highly effective in treating pain, inflammation and swelling that often come with tonsillitis. Popsicles and ice chips can be particularly helpful to young children who can't use other home remedies safely.

- Humidifiers; humidifiers can help to relieve the sore throat if the air is dry or you are experiencing dry mouth as a result of tonsillitis.

HOME REMEDY FOR LOSS OF SMELL (ANOSMIA)

The following dietary ingredients can help improve loss of sense of smell;

- ❖ Castor oil
- ❖ Garlic
- ❖ Ginger
- ❖ Cayenne pepper

- ❖ Lemon

- ❖ Apple cidar vinegar

- ❖ Cinnamon

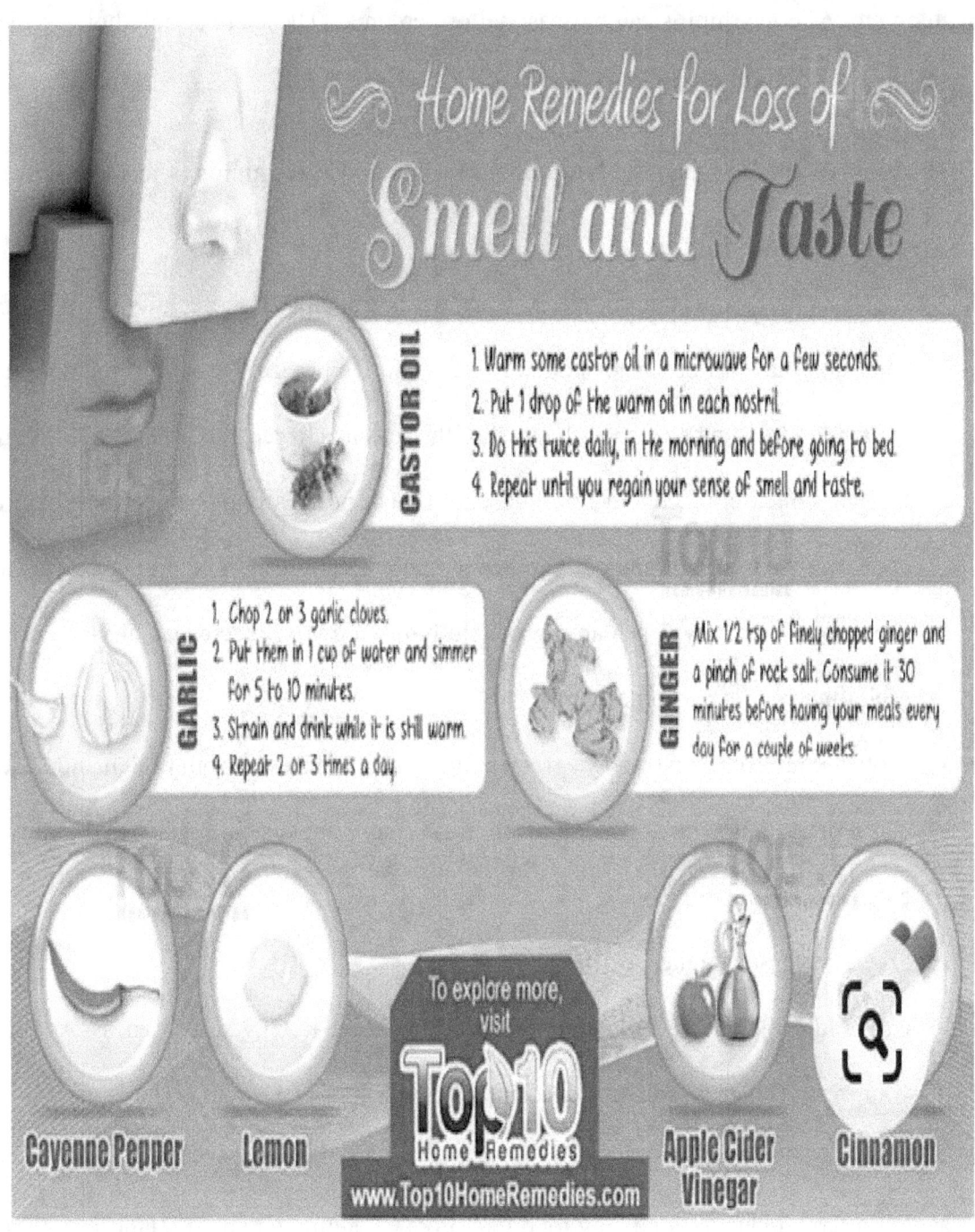

HOME REMEDIES FOR SEASONAL ALLERGIC RHINITIS

An allergen is an otherwise harmless substance that can cause an allergic reaction. Allergic rhinitis is an allergic response to specific allergens such as pollen, dust, animal dander, detergents etc. This response produces symptoms such as running nose, sneezing, stuffy nose, itchy nose, watery nose, coughing etc. Allergic rhinitis can be seasonal or perennial. These are simple home remedies for seasonal rhinitis;

- ➤ Avoid allergy triggers; the best way to manage allergic rhinitis is to identify the allergy triggers and avoid them.

- ➤ Allergy-proof your house; Keep your windows closed, especially when warm, dry condition makes it easier for pollen to travel on the breeze. Be sure to put aclean filter in the air conditioning system at the start of the season and replaced it every 2-3 months.

- ➤ Reduce pollen cling; like a fine household dust, pollens clings to clothes, skin and just about anything else it lands on. To reduce pollen clings, avoid hanging clothes, towel or sheets outside to dry. Use damp wash cloth to wipe your face especially around the eyes each time you return home.

- ➤ Protect your eyes; wearing eye glasses can protect your eyes from pollen and dust.

- ➤ Nasal irrigation with saline solution flushes out mucus, allergens and relieves nasal congestion.

- ➤ Stay away from smoke.

- ➤ Use cold compresses; cold compress can help reduce itching and soreness. Avoid rubbing your eyes. This makes itching and irritation worse.

- ➤ Drink plenty of water.

- ➤ Eat allergy reducing food; any food that produce natural and high quantities of vitamin C, zinc, vitamin D, antioxidants and other helpful vitamin and minerals (blueberries, apples, onions, honey etc) can boost the immune system and are good choices for fighting nasal allergies.

VERTIGO; is a feeling of spinning sensation. It is caused by your senses telling your brain that your body is off balance, even though it isn't.

HOME MANAGEMENT OF VERTIGO

- ✓ Stress management; some conditions that cause vertigo, including Meniere's disease, can be triggered by stress. Developing coping strategies to navigate stressful circumstances could decrease your episodes of vertigo. Practicing meditation and deep breathing techniques are a good place to start.

- ✓ Adequate amount of sleep; feelings of vertigo can be triggered by sleep deprivation. If you are experiencing vertigo for the first time, it might be a result of stress or lack of sleep.

- ✓ Avoiding alcohol; beyond the dizziness you feel while drinking, alcohol can actually change the composition of the fluid in your inner ear. Alcohol also dehydrate you. These things can affect your balance even when you are sober.

- ✓ Hydration; sometimes vertigo is caused by simple dehydration. Reducing sodium intake may help. But the best way to stay hydrated is to drink plenty of water.

- ✓ Vitamin D; if you suspect your vertigo is connected to something you aren't getting in your diet, you could be right. Lack of vitamin D can worsen symptoms for people that have BPPV, the most common cause of vertigo. A glass of fortified milk, canned tuna and even egg yolk will give your vitamin D level a boost.

✓ Ginko biloba; the use of ginko biloba can be effective in managing vertigo and tinnitus as well. Ginko biloba extract can be purchased in liquid or capsule form.

✓ Epley maneuver; Epley maneuver is a vestibular exercise that can be effective in relieving your vertigo. You can perform this maneuver at home by following this simple procedure;

1. Start by sitting upright on a flat surface with a pillow behind you and with your legs outstretched.

2. Turn your head 45 degrees to the right.

3. With your head still tilted, quickly recline with your head on the pillow. Stay in this position for at least 30 seconds.

4. Slowly turn your head to the left, a full 90 degrees, without lifting your neck.

5. Engage your whole body, turning it to the left so that you are completely on your left side.

6. Slowly turn to your original position, looking forward and sitting straight up. You can have someone assist with epley maneuver by guiding your head according to the steps outlined above.

See image below

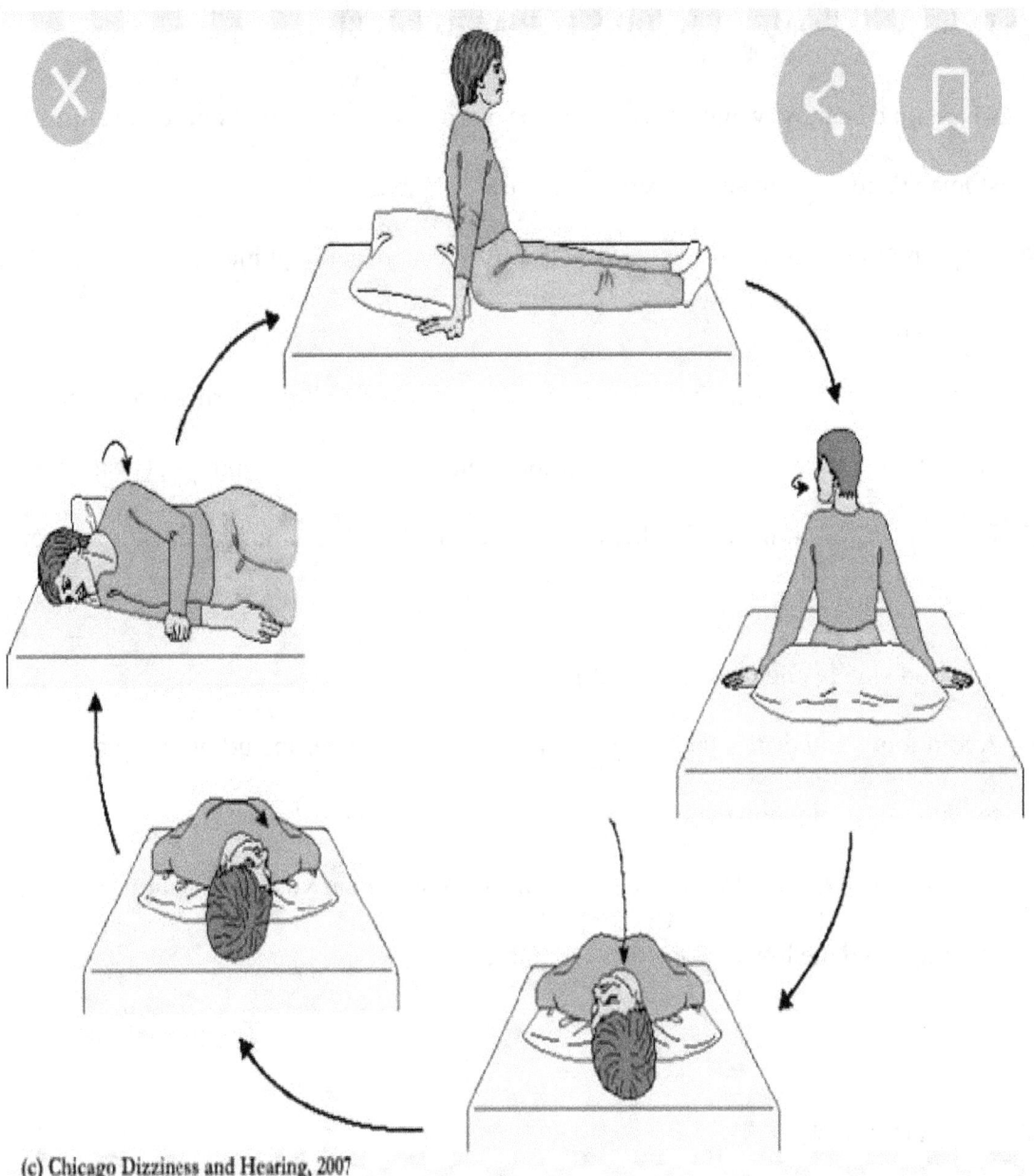

(c) Chicago Dizziness and Hearing, 2007

LIFESTYLE AND HOME REMEDIES FOR ACID REFLUX

❖ Maintain a healthy weight; excess pounds put pressure on your abdomen, pushing up your stomach and causing acid to reflux into your esophagus.

❖ Stop smoking; smoking decreases the lower esophageal sphincter's ability to function properly.

❖ Elevate the head of your bed; if you regularly experience heart burn while trying to sleep, elevate the head end of your bed in order to elevate your body from your waist up.

❖ Don't lie down immediately after a meal; wait at least three hours after eating before lying or going to bed.

❖ Eat food slowly and chew thoroughly.

❖ Avoid foods and drinks that trigger reflux; common trigger including, fatty or fried foods, tomato sauce, alcohol, chocolate, mint, garlic, onion and caffeine.

❖ Avoid tight-fighting clothing; clothes that fit tight around your waist put pressure on your abdomen and the lower esophageal sphincter.

LIVING WITH TINNITUS

Tinnitus is the ringing, hissing, or buzzing sounds in your ears that other people don't hear. Tinnitus can be very disturbing and may affect your daily activities. These approaches should be used along with any treatments or hearing aids suggested by your doctor.

Learn what makes tinnitus worse for you. Some people report that certain foods, drinks, or drugs can make their symptoms worse. Not everyone is affected the same way, so try to avoid triggers one at a time and keep a written log.

Some possible triggers include:

Drinks with caffeine such as cola, coffee, tea, and energy drinks

- Alcohol
- AspirinSalt

These are Simple Ways that May Help In Dealing With Your Tinnitus.

1. Kick the habit, if you smoke.Smoking can make tinnitus worse in two ways. It harms blood flow to the sensitive nerve cells that control your hearing.

2. Add soothing sounds to silence. Tinnitus may bother you more when it's quiet. So try these tips to distract yourself from the ringing in your ears:

- ➤ Play soft music in the background
- ➤ Listen to the radio
- ➤ Turn on a fan

3. Plan time to relax every day. It's normal to feel anxious and annoyed when you first develop tinnitus or when it flares up. But stress and worry can make your symptoms worse.Try these relaxation methods:

- ➤ Yoga
- ➤ Tai-chi
- ➤ Meditation
- ➤ Progressive muscle relaxation

4. Get enough sleep. Fatigue often makes symptoms worse, turning a soft hum into a loud roar. If tinnitus keeps you from sleeping well, this can become a vicious cycle.Practice good sleep habits for more restful sleep:

- Make your bedroom dark and cool.

- Use a fan or white-noise machine if your bedroom is too quiet.

- Set aside 7 to 9 hours for sleep at night.

- Go to bed and get up at the same time every day.

- Develop a bedtime routine, such as taking a relaxing warm bath right before bedtime.

- Make sure your bed and pillows are comfortable and supportive.

5. Join a support group. Talking with other people with the same condition can help you feel less alone. You'll also learn different approaches for coping with tinnitus.

6. Protect your hearing. Loud noise is a common cause of tinnitus. It can also make your symptoms worse for a short time.

Here are some ways to protect yourself from our noisy world:

- Keep music at 60% of full volume or lower when using earbuds. Don't listen for more than 60 minutes at one time.

- Wear ear plugs at concerts, loud restaurants, or other loud events. If you can't hear someone standing an arm's length away, it's loud enough to cause hearing damage and make tinnitus worse.

- Use ear plugs or earmuffs when cutting the grass, using power tools, or using snow or leaf blowers.

- Always use ear protection in a noisy place.

7. If tinnitus persist, consult your doctor or ENT practitioner. Your tinnitus may be caused by the following disorders:

- ➢ Thyroid disorders

- ➢ High blood pressure

- ➢ Lyme disease

- ➢ Fibromyalgia

- ➢ Ear wax buildup

- ➢ Jaw misalignment

- ➢ Traumatic brain injury

- ➢ Stroke

- ➢ Diabetes

CHOKING RESCUE FOR BABIES

WARNING: Do not begin the choking rescue procedure unless you are certain that the baby is choking. If a baby can't breathe, cough, or make sounds, then:

- ➢ Put the baby face down on your forearm so the baby's head is lower than his or her chest.

- ➢ Support the baby's head in your palm, against your thigh. Don't cover the baby's mouth or twist his or her neck.

- ➢ Use the heel of one hand to give up to 5 back slaps between the baby's shoulder blades. See picture A.

- ➢ If the object does not pop out, support the baby's head and turn him or her faceup on your thigh. Keep the baby's head lower than his or her body.

- Place 2 or 3 fingers just below the nipple line on the baby's breastbone and give 5 quick chest thrusts (same position as chest compressions in CPR for a baby). See picture B.

- Keep giving 5 back slaps and 5 chest thrusts until the object comes out or the baby faints.

- If the baby faints, then,

- Do not do any more back slaps or chest thrusts.

- Start CPR. If you do rescue breaths, look for an object in the mouth or throat each time the airway is opened during CPR. If you see the object, take it out. But if you can't see the object, don't stick your finger down the baby's throat to feel for it.

- Keep doing CPR until the baby is breathing on his or her own or until help arrive

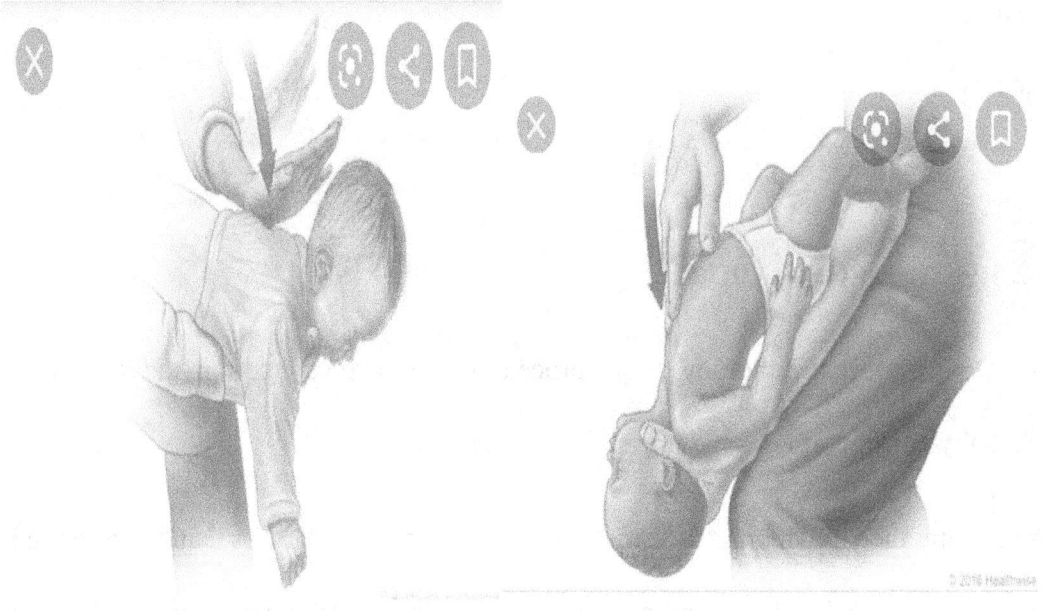

Picture B. CPR for babies

SIMPLE WAYS OF MANAGING SNORING

To prevent or quiet snoring, try these tips:

1. If you're overweight, lose weight.

2. Sleep on your side.

3. Raise the head of your bed.

4. Nasal strips or an external nasal dilator.

5. Treat nasal congestion or obstruction.

6. Limit or avoid alcohol and sedatives.

7. Quit smoking.

8. Get enough sleep.

DEALING WITH DROOLING OF SALIVA

Drooling is expected in babies, who do not yet have full control over their mouths or swallowing muscles. But drooling is often embarrassing for children and adults. Many people may avoid discussing this symptom.

Drooling can occur for many reasons. Most people drool every once in a while. It is especially common while sleeping, when a person swallows less frequently. This can cause saliva to accumulate and seep from the sides of the mouth.

For those wondering how to stop drooling, the best method may depend on the cause.

The best ways to stop drooling include;

1. Change sleeping position: If a person is drooling while asleep, switching to sleeping on the back may be a quick fix. Gravity will prevent saliva from seeping out of the mouth. A wedge pillow can help a person to stay in one position all night.

2. Treat allergies and sinus problems. Sinus infections and allergies can lead to increased saliva production and a stuffy nose. Having a blocked nose causes a person to breathe through the mouth, making it easier for saliva to escape.

3. Take medication. A doctor may recommend medicine to eliminate drooling, especially in patients with neurological conditions. Scopolamine, also known as hyoscine, intercepts nerve impulses before they reach the salivary glands. This medication is often delivered in the form of a patch placed behind the ear. The patch releases the medication continuously, and one patch typically lasts for about 72 hours. Side effects of scopolamine may include: dizziness, drowsiness, an increased heart rate, dry mouth, itchy eyes. Glycopyrrolate is another option. It also decreases saliva production by blocking nerve impulses, but side effects can be more severe. They may include: irritability, trouble urinating, hyperactivity, skin flushing, decreased sweating

4. .Receive Botox injections. Botox injections in the salivary glands may help to prevent drooling. Botulinum toxin (Botox) injections have been used to treat drooling in people with neurological disorders. A doctor injects Botox into the salivary glands, usually with the assistance of ultrasound imaging. The Botox paralyzes the muscles in the area, preventing the salivary glands from functioning.

5. Attend speech therapy. Depending on the cause of drooling, a doctor may recommend speech therapy. The goal is to improve jaw stability and tongue strength and mobility.

This therapy can also help a person to close the lips fully. Speech therapy may take time, but a person can learn techniques to improve swallowing and decrease drooling.

6. Use an oral appliance. An oral appliance is a device placed in the mouth to assist with swallowing. The device helps with tongue positioning and lip closure. When a person is better able to swallow, they are likely to drool less.

Change sleeping positions

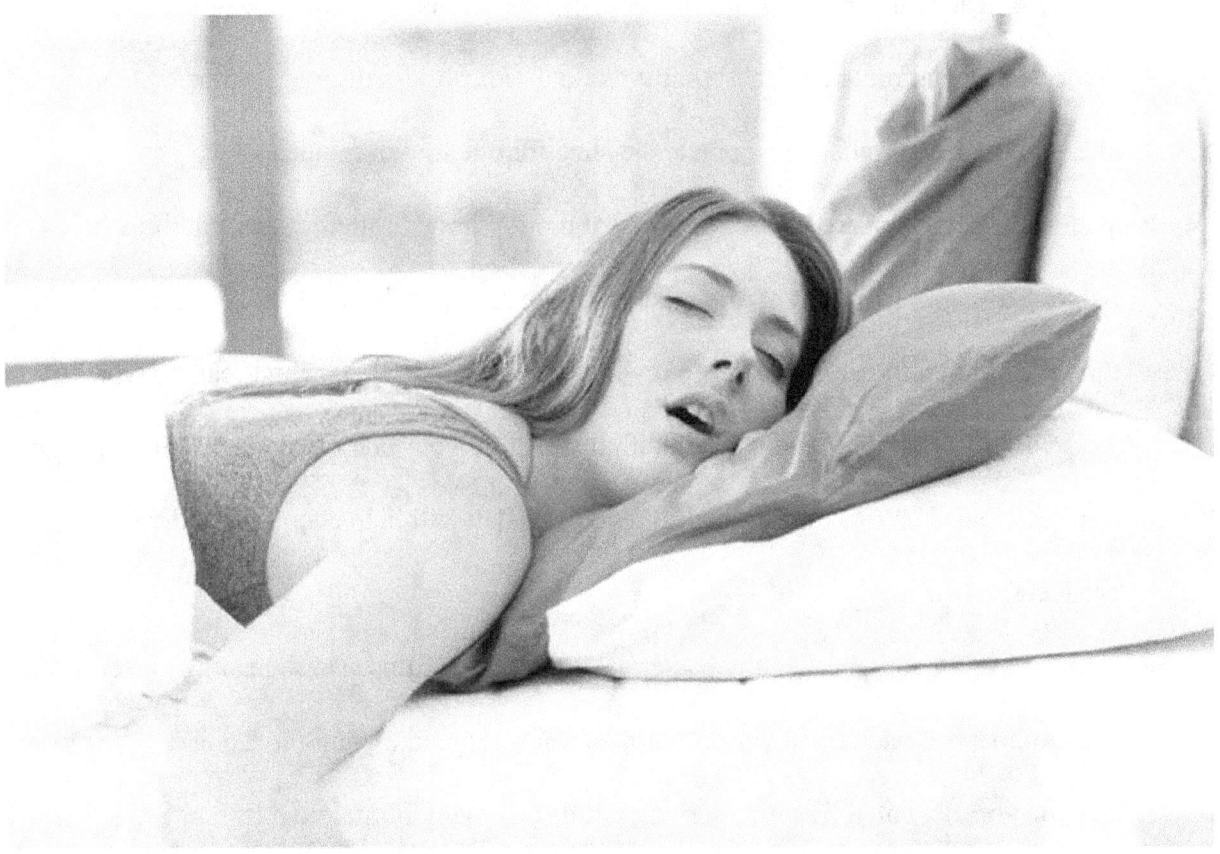

Certain sleeping positions may encourage drooling.

HOME REMEDIES FOR BAD BREATH (HALITOSI)

❖ Good dental hygiene: According to research studies Trusted Source, poor dental hygiene is the most common cause of bad breath. Preventing plaque buildup is the key to maintaining a healthy mouth. You should brush your teeth using a fluoride toothpaste for two minutes at least twice per day (morning and night).

❖ Parsley: Parsley is a popular folk remedy for bad breath. Its fresh scent and high chlorophyll content suggest that it can have a deodorizing effect.

❖ Pineapple juice: Many people believe that pineapple juice is the quickest and most effective treatment for bad breath. While there is no scientific evidence to back up this theory, anecdotal reports suggest that it works.Drink a glass of organic pineapple juice after every meal, or chew on a pineapple slice for one to two minutes.

❖ Water: Research Trusted Source shows that mouth dryness often causes bad breath. Saliva plays a very important role in keeping your mouth clean. Without it, bacteria thrive. Your mouth naturally dries out while you sleep, which is why breath is typically worse in the morning. Prevent dry mouth by keeping your body hydrated. Drinking water (not caffeinated or sugary drinks) throughout the day will help encourage saliva production.

❖ Yogurt: Yogurt contains healthy bacteria called lactobacillus. These healthy bacteria can help combat bad bacteria in various parts of your body, like your gut. To use yogurt to fight bad breath, eat at least one serving per day of plain, nonfat yogurt.

❖ Milk: Milk is a well-known cure for bad breath. Research shows that drinking milk after eating garlic can significantly improve "garlicky" breath. To use this method, drink a glass of low- or full-fat milk during or after a meal containing strong-smelling foods like garlic and onions.

❖ Zinc: Zinc salts, an ingredient in certain mouthwashesTrusted Source and chewing gumTrusted Source, can counteract bad breath. Zinc works to decrease the number of sulfurous compounds in your breath.Try a zinc chewing gum designed for people with dry mouth. You can also find zinc dietary supplements at your local drug store.

❖ Homemade mouthwash with vinegar: Vinegar contains a natural acid called acetic acid. Bacteria don't like to grow in acidic environments, so a vinegar mouthwash may reduce bacteria growth. Add 2 tablespoons of white or apple cider vinegar to 1 cup of water. Gargle for at least 30 seconds before spitting it out.

CONCLUSION

In conclusion, most ear, nose, and throat problems can be managed without medication at home. This can help reduce cost and time spent at health care facilities. However, severe ear, nose and throat (ENT) conditions should be reported to the ENT specialist for urgent treatment.

www.ingramcontent.com/pod-product-compliance
Lightning Source LLC
Chambersburg PA
CBHW080630220526
45467CB00011B/3458